ALISTAIR PEDLOW

Living With Ankylosis Spondylitis And Cancer

Accomplishing Life With Ankylosis Spondylitis & Cancer

This book was professionally typeset on Reedsy.
Find out more at reedsy.com

1

Forward

Welcome to my book, "Living with Ankylosis Spondylitis and Cancer." I am excited to share my journey with you. This book is a reflection of my personal experiences living with two chronic and life-changing diseases, Ankylosis Spondylitis (AS) and prostate cancer.

AS is a rare autoimmune disease that affects the spine and joints, causing pain, stiffness, and loss of mobility. Prostate cancer, on the other hand, is a common form of cancer that affects men and can have a range of outcomes depending on when it is detected and treated.

When I was first diagnosed with AS, I felt overwhelmed and scared. I was in my early 50s and had already been dealing with the symptoms for decades without knowing what was causing them. It was only after a car accident and an MRI that I was diagnosed with AS. The diagnosis was a relief in some ways, as I finally had a name for what I was experiencing. However, it was also a shock to learn that I had a rare autoimmune disease with no cure.

Living with AS meant adjusting my lifestyle to manage the symptoms. I had to learn how to manage the pain, stiffness, and mobility issues while still maintaining an active and fulfilling life. It was a challenging journey, but I learned a lot about myself and the importance of self-care.

Just when I thought I had found my rhythm living with AS, I was diagnosed with prostate cancer. This was a completely different experience from AS. I had to navigate the medical system and make decisions about my treatment options. There were moments of fear, doubt, and uncertainty, but I learned to trust my gut instincts and advocate for myself.

Living with these two chronic diseases was not easy, but it taught me a lot about resilience, self-care, and the importance of community. Through my experiences, I have gained valuable insights into living with chronic illness, and I hope to share these lessons with you in this book.

I will share my journey with AS and prostate cancer, including the challenges I faced and the lessons I learned along the way. I will provide practical advice and tips for managing the symptoms of AS and navigating the medical system. I will also discuss the emotional toll of living with chronic illness and the importance of community support.

This book is not just for those living with AS and prostate cancer, but also for anyone living with other chronic illnesses. I hope that my journey will inspire and empower others to take control of their health and find ways to live fulfilling lives despite these conditions.

Thank you for joining me on this journey, and I hope you find this book to be a valuable resource and source of inspiration.

2

Introduction

My name is Aili Williams and I am looking forward to sharing my experience living with my disease. I am fifty-five years old as I write this book, and I have been living with both conditions for the last four years. The story goes way back many years before I was diagnosed with Ankylosis Spondylitis in 2018 and then in 2019 with Prostate Cancer.

This book is my experiences a mix of good and bad as I migrated my way through the changes in my life with Ankylosis Spondylitis & prostate cancer. I will document my care plan, medication and operations for my prostate cancer over the four years. There were many added difficulties and challenges due to the Covid-19 pandemic and how that framed the first two years of my NHS treatment and the care I needed. We will cover the emotional impact and exhausting physical experiences I faced as I began this journey into the unknown.

As I got older, I noticed that my body was not functioning as it should. My joints were stiff and painful, and I had difficulty moving around. I found that I was unable to do things that I used to take for granted, like

3

bending down to tie my shoelaces or reaching for something on a high shelf. I attributed these issues to ageing, but the truth was much more complicated.

It wasn't until I had an MRI after a car accident back in the late 80s that it was suggested that I may have a condition called Ankylosing Spondylitis. Ankylosing Spondylitis is a chronic inflammatory disease that primarily affects the spine and other joints, causing pain, stiffness and loss of mobility. Although it is a relatively rare condition, it can cause significant disability if not properly managed.

My diagnosis came as a shock to me, as I had never heard of Ankylosing Spondylitis before. I was fortunate to have a supportive medical team who provided me with information about the condition and helped me to understand what it meant for my future. However, I also discovered that not all medical professionals are equally knowledgeable about rare conditions like Ankylosing Spondylitis.

As I navigated the medical system, I learned the importance of advocating for myself and being well-informed about my condition. I read everything I could find about Ankylosing Spondylitis and joined support groups where I could connect with others who were living with the same condition. I also sought second opinions when unsure about a particular treatment or medication.

One of the challenges of living with Ankylosing Spondylitis is that it is a progressive disease that can lead to complications like spinal fusion, eye inflammation and heart problems. However, I found that by staying informed about my condition and being proactive about my healthcare, I was able to manage my symptoms and maintain a good quality of life.

Life threw another curveball at me when I was diagnosed with prostate cancer in my early 50s. Although the diagnosis was a shock, I felt more prepared to navigate the medical system this time around. I had learned the importance of being well-informed and advocating for myself, and I was better equipped to understand the different treatment options that were available to me.

Prostate cancer is a common type of cancer that affects the prostate gland, which is located in the male reproductive system. It is the second most common type of cancer in men worldwide, with over 1 million new cases diagnosed each year.

My diagnosis was caught early through routine screening, which is recommended for men over the age of 50. Although the diagnosis was scary, I was fortunate to have a supportive medical team who helped me to understand my options and provided me with the information I needed to make informed decisions about my care.

One of the biggest challenges of living with prostate cancer was managing the side effects of treatment, including urinary incontinence and erectile dysfunction, however, I found that by being open and honest with my medical team, I was able to receive the support and resources I needed to manage these issues.

Through my experience with Ankylosing Spondylitis and prostate cancer, I have learned the importance of being an active participant in my healthcare. By staying informed about my condition and advocating for myself, I have been able to maintain a good quality of life and manage my symptoms effectively.

For others who may be facing similar health challenges, my advice is to always trust your instincts and listen to your body. If something doesn't feel right, don't be afraid to ask questions and seek out additional information. Connect with others who are living with similar conditions and join support groups to find the resources and support you need. Finally, remember that you are not alone and that there is always hope for a better tomorrow.

As a non-medical person, the information and resources I share will be from my own experiences and should not be taken as being something you should do as a reader. I will discuss how I met the changes and challenges medically with my medical teams who didn't always get it right.

I hope this book will inspire you to achieve your full potential even though the odds are stacked against you. Life will continue to be challenging; however, we must always strive to be the best versions of ourselves as we can be no matter what.

Living with Ankylosing Spondylitis (AS) and cancer can be a challenging experience that can impact a person's physical, emotional, and social well-being. AS is a chronic condition that primarily affects the spine and other joints in the body, while cancer is a group of diseases characterized by the uncontrolled growth and spread of abnormal cells.

AS can cause pain, stiffness, reduced mobility, and fatigue, which can make it difficult to perform daily activities. Cancer, on the other hand, can cause a range of symptoms depending on the location and stage of cancer, as well as the type of treatment received. Cancer treatments such as chemotherapy and radiation therapy can also worsen AS symptoms, making it even more challenging to manage both conditions.

Living with both AS and cancer requires a comprehensive approach to treatment that takes into account the unique challenges of managing both conditions. This may involve working closely with a healthcare team that includes specialists in both AS and cancer, developing a personalized treatment plan that addresses the needs of both conditions, and managing symptoms such as pain, fatigue, and nausea.

Maintaining a healthy lifestyle, including regular exercise, a balanced diet, and stress management techniques, can also help manage both AS and cancer. Emotional support from family, friends, and support groups also play a very important role in managing the challenges of living with both conditions.

Living with both AS and cancer can be challenging, it is important to remember there are ways to manage both conditions and maintain a good quality of life. We need to work closely with healthcare providers, manage symptoms, and maintain a healthy lifestyle. Those of us with AS and cancer can live fulfilling lives despite the limitations of both diseases.

3

So what is it like to live with Ankylosis Spondylitis (AS)

Ankylosing Spondylitis is a type of arthritis that primarily affects the spine, causing inflammation, stiffness, and pain. It can also affect other joints, such as the hips and shoulders, elbows, knees and ankles. AS is a chronic condition that can lead to complications such as decreased mobility, spinal fusion, and deformity.

The first sign that something was wrong was when I started to have bouts of Iritis, around my mid to late thirties. Iritis, also known as anterior uveitis, is an inflammation of the iris and other structures in the front of the eye. It is a type of uveitis, which refers to inflammation of the uvea, the middle layer of the eye.

The symptoms of iritis may include eye pain, redness, sensitivity to light (photophobia), blurred vision, and a small pupil that doesn't respond to changes in light. Iritis can be caused by a variety of factors, including autoimmune disorders (AS), infections, injuries to the eye, or as a side effect of certain medications.

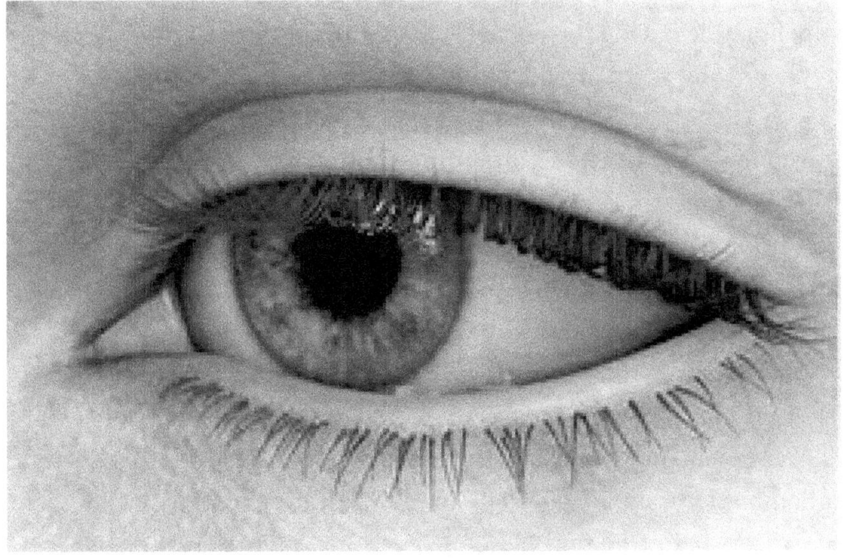

Iritis

Treatment for iritis typically involves using eye drops that contain corticosteroids to reduce inflammation and relieve symptoms. In some cases, other medications or procedures may be necessary, depending on the underlying cause of the iritis. It is important to seek medical attention if you experience any symptoms of iritis, as it can lead to complications such as glaucoma or cataracts if left untreated.

I felt like I had been hit with a baseball bat on the side of the head, the pain was unbearable. My left eye looked like a blue steak, inflamed and angry. I had to wear sunglass as my eyes were extremely sensitive to the light, this added to the discomfort and pain. I was sent to the emergency room by my General practitioner (GP), as I have outlined this condition can have long-lasting problems if not treated promptly. I was given medication and sent on my way, with no follow-up as to why I may be having this issue. This was one of the first mistakes made by the medical care provided in my region.

It would not be until 2017, after my tenth bout of iritis, and a relocation to a different country, I would be asked if I had been tested for a condition called Ankylosing Spondylitis (HLA-B27) gene. My blood test came back positive for the defective gene, which answered a lot of questions about how and why I felt the way I did.

One possible reason for the increased cancer risk in people with AS is the chronic inflammation that occurs in the body. Chronic inflammation can damage cells and DNA, leading to the development of cancer. Additionally, some medications used to treat AS, such as nonsteroidal anti-inflammatory drugs (NSAIDs), may increase the risk of cancer.

If you have AS and are concerned about your cancer risk, it is important to talk to your doctor. They can evaluate your risk and recommend appropriate screening tests or other preventative measures.

If you have been diagnosed with cancer and have AS, your treatment options may be affected. For example, some cancer treatments can worsen AS symptoms, such as spinal fusion. Your healthcare team can work with you to develop a treatment plan that takes into account both your cancer and AS.

In summary, while there may be a possible link between AS and cancer, more research is needed to fully understand the relationship between the two. If you have AS and are concerned about your cancer risk, talk to your doctor about your options. If you have been diagnosed with cancer and have AS, work with your healthcare team to develop a treatment plan that takes both conditions into account.

AS Linked with other diseases

Ankylosing Spondylitis (AS) is a type of arthritis that primarily affects the spine, but can also affect other joints in the body. It is a chronic condition that can lead to complications such as decreased mobility, spinal fusion, and deformity. AS is also associated with other related diseases and conditions.

Some of the related diseases and conditions associated with AS include:

1. Inflammatory bowel disease (IBD): IBD is a group of disorders that cause chronic inflammation of the digestive tract. There is a strong association between AS and IBD, with up to 50% of people with AS also having IBD.
2. Psoriasis: Psoriasis is a chronic skin condition that causes red, scaly patches on the skin. People with AS are more likely to have psoriasis than the general population.
3. Uveitis: Uveitis is an inflammation of the eye that can cause pain, redness, and vision loss. About 25% of people with AS will develop uveitis at some point in their lives.
4. Osteoporosis: Osteoporosis is a condition in which the bones become weak and brittle, making them more prone to fractures. People with AS are at an increased risk of developing osteoporosis due to decreased mobility and the use of certain medications.
5. Cardiovascular disease: People with AS are at an increased risk of developing cardiovascular diseases, such as heart attack and stroke. This may be due to chronic inflammation and the effect of AS on the blood vessels.
6. Depression and anxiety: People with chronic conditions like AS

may be at an increased risk of developing depression and anxiety.

7. Fatigue: Fatigue is a common symptom of AS, and it can be debilitating for some people.

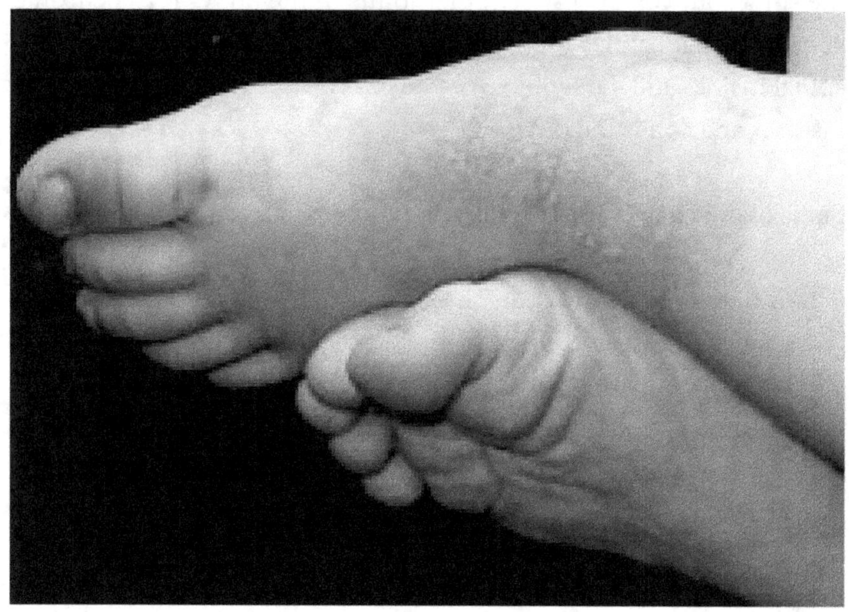

Psoriasis

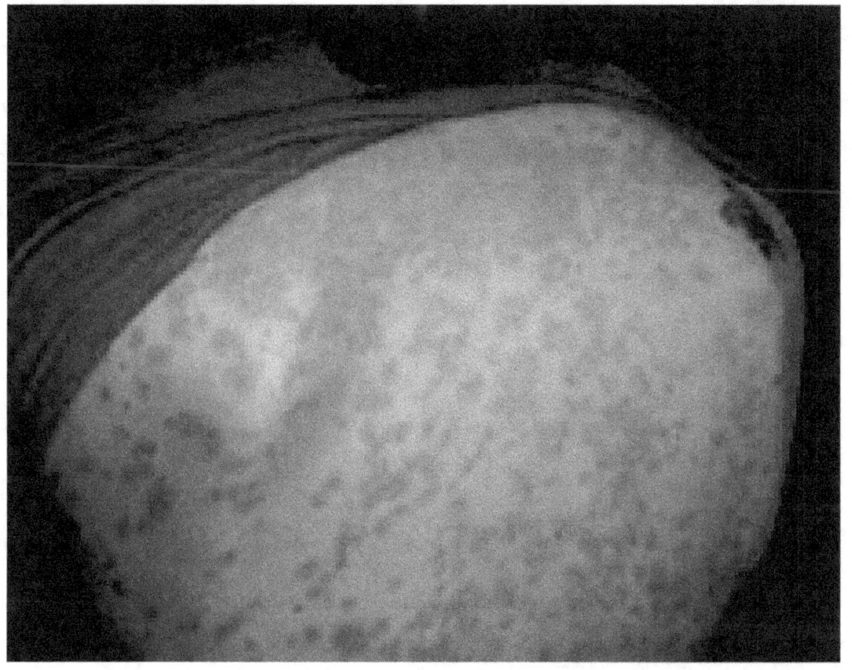

Psoriasis

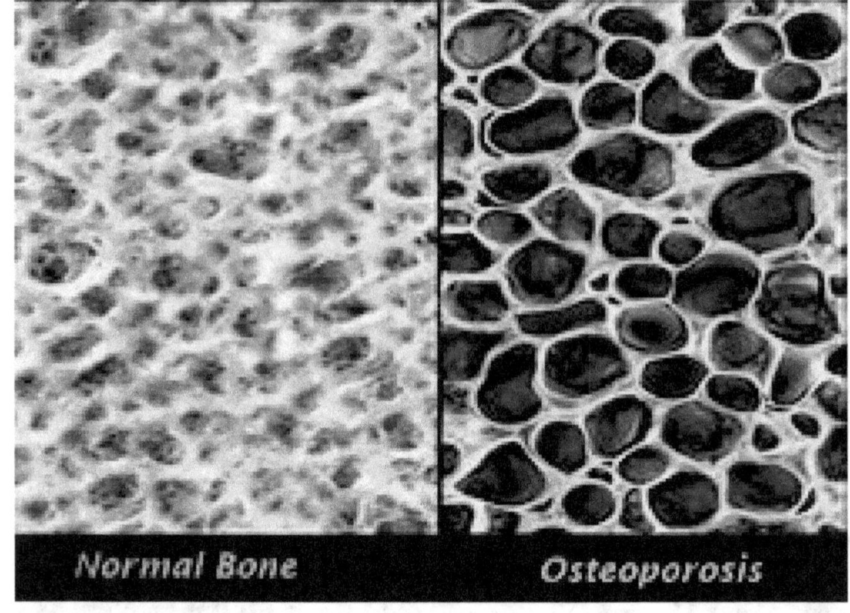

Osteoporosis

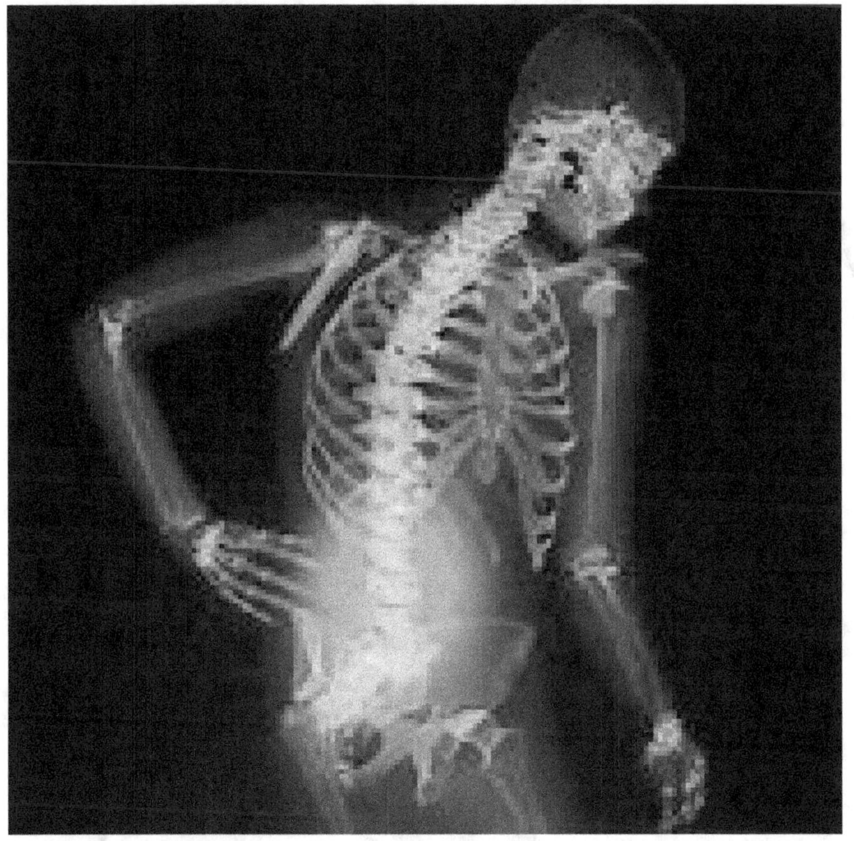

Osteoporosis

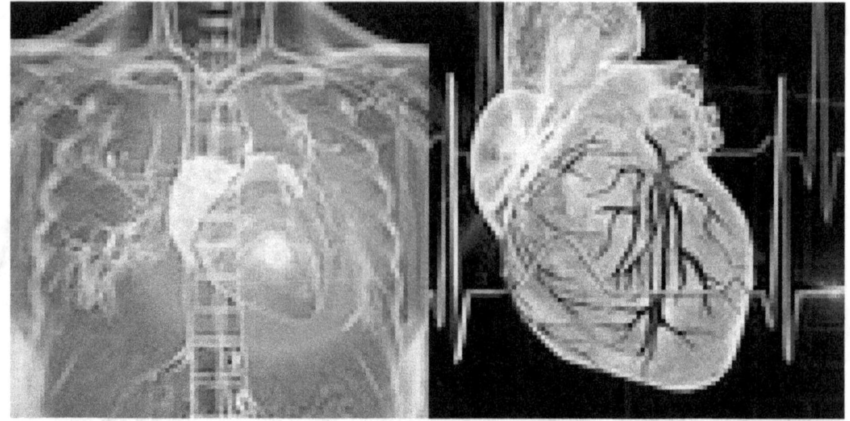

Cardiovascular disease

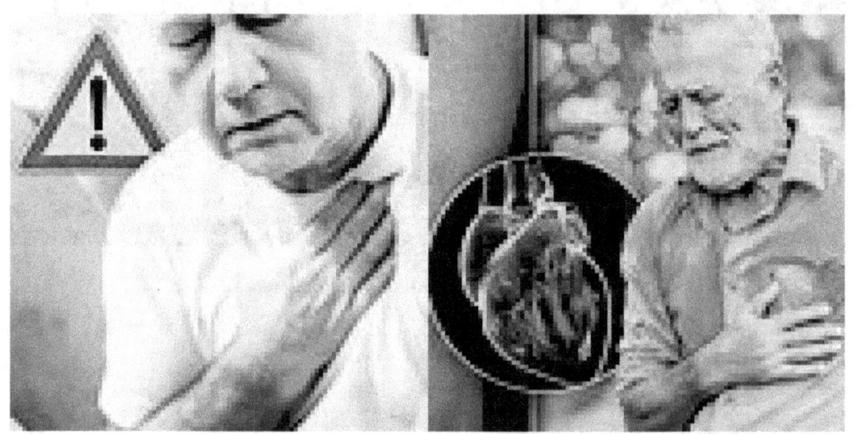

Cardiovascular disease

Overall, AS is associated with several related diseases and conditions, and people with AS need to receive regular medical care and screening for these conditions. By managing these related conditions, people with AS can improve their overall health and quality of life.

Ankylosing Spondylitis (AS) usually starts in early adulthood, typically between the ages of 20 and 40. However, AS can develop at any age, including during childhood and later in life.

The onset of AS can be gradual, with symptoms developing over months or years. In some cases, symptoms can appear suddenly. AS affects men more often than women, and it has a genetic component, meaning it runs in families.

If you have a family history of AS or are experiencing symptoms such as back pain and stiffness, pain and stiffness in other joints, and fatigue, talk to your doctor. Early diagnosis and treatment can help manage symptoms and slow the progression of the disease.

Living with Ankylosing Spondylitis (AS) and cancer can be a challenging experience that can impact a person's physical, emotional, and social well-being. AS is a chronic condition that primarily affects the spine and other joints in the body, while cancer is a group of diseases characterised by the uncontrolled growth and spread of abnormal cells.

AS can cause pain, stiffness, reduced mobility, and fatigue, which can make it difficult to perform daily activities. Cancer, on the other hand, can cause a range of symptoms depending on the location and stage of cancer, as well as the type of treatment received. Cancer treatments such as chemotherapy and radiation therapy can also worsen AS symptoms, making it even more challenging to manage both conditions.

Living with both AS and cancer requires a comprehensive approach to treatment that takes into account the unique challenges of managing both conditions. This may involve working closely with a healthcare team that includes specialists in both AS and cancer, developing a personalized treatment plan that addresses the needs of both conditions, and managing symptoms such as pain, fatigue, and nausea.

Maintaining a healthy lifestyle, including regular exercise, a balanced diet, and stress management techniques, can also help manage both AS and cancer. Emotional support from family, friends, and support groups can also help manage the challenges of living with both conditions.

While living with both AS and cancer can be challenging, it is important to remember that there are ways to manage both conditions and maintain a good quality of life. By working closely with healthcare providers, managing symptoms, and maintaining a healthy lifestyle, people with AS and cancer can live fulfilling lives despite the challenges of managing both conditions.

There have been many studies conducted on Ankylosing Spondylitis (AS) over the years, to better understand the condition and develop effective treatments. Here are some examples of studies conducted on AS:

1. Genetic studies: AS is known to have a genetic component, and researchers have identified several genes that are associated with the condition. These studies have helped to shed light on the underlying mechanisms of AS and may lead to new treatments in the future.
2. Imaging studies: Imaging techniques such as X-rays, CT scans, and MRI scans have been used to study the changes that occur in the spine and other joints in people with AS. These studies have helped to improve the diagnosis and monitoring of the condition.
3. Clinical trials: Clinical trials are studies that test new treatments or therapies in people with a particular condition. Several

clinical trials have been conducted on AS, testing drugs such as nonsteroidal anti-inflammatory drugs (NSAIDs), biologics, and other therapies. These studies have helped to identify effective treatments for AS.

4. Epidemiological studies: Epidemiological studies are studies that examine the incidence and prevalence of a particular condition in a population. Several epidemiological studies have been conducted on AS, helping to better understand the demographics of the condition and identify risk factors.

5. Quality of life studies: AS can have a significant impact on a person's quality of life, and researchers have outlined some of the limiting factors in a person's life with AS.

Initially, my overwhelming issue with AS was chronic fatigue and trying to get through my working day and home life. I would wake in the morning feeling as if I had never been to bed. My job required me to travel a lot with work which involved a lot of driving. I recall leaving home to go to a work location, only to get halfway and I would have to pull into a service stop and rest before I could continue. There were many occasions when I had to return home as it was impossible to continue with my day.

I was assigned a Rheumatologist to find out the impact this was having on my body and possible treatments I may need to aid in living with this incurable disease. I went through many tests, including blood tests, X-rays, MRIs and many others. I was prescribed many different painkillers to help manage the symptoms and pain, however; to no avail. As I mentioned many other conditions go along with AS, depression being one of them. Living with any chronic condition on a long-term base can cause mental fatigue and in my case did. I was diagnosed in

2018/19 with clinical depression and prescribed medication. It is very easy to spiral out of control, falling into a perpetual cycle of pain and depression.

I would strongly advise seeking medical help from your doctor if you feel your condition is causing anxiety and depression, the quicker you can do this the better. As we have mentioned it is very common for anyone with a long-term illness to experience anxiety and depression. In my experience, the more you can verbalise what impacts the condition has on your life the better, this may just help you come to terms with what you can not control. I am always on the lookout for any like-minded groups, I could join where I could ask the questions I needed, and express my concerns with people that fully understood what I was experiencing. These can be local groups or groups online (Facebook) which helped me to realise I was not alone in my fight. I found the Ankylosing Spondylitis Society.

By late 2019, my condition had worsened to the point I was unable to work or function daily at home. My Rheumatologist suggested we could consider (biological injection therapy treatment). My doctor when through the treatment plan I could go with, and also the potential side effects you can experience while on this treatment. At this point in my condition, I would have tried anything. While this treatment is not a cure, it can slow the progression of your disease.

Biological treatments for AS are generally reserved for patients who have not responded well to other therapies, such as nonsteroidal anti-inflammatory drugs (NSAIDs) and disease-modifying antirheumatic drugs (DMARDs). They can be highly effective in reducing inflammation and improving symptoms, but they can also have side effects, such as an increased risk of infections. Therefore, it is important to discuss the potential risks and benefits of these medications with your healthcare provider.

4

What is Biological Therapy Treatment?

Biological treatments, also known as biologics or biologic response modifiers, are a type of medication that can be used to treat AS.

Biological treatments for AS target specific molecules in the immune system that are involved in inflammation, such as tumour necrosis factor-alpha (TNF-alpha), interleukin-17 (IL-17), and interleukin-23 (IL-23). These medications are usually given by injection or infusion, and they work by blocking the activity of these molecules, which helps to reduce inflammation and alleviate symptoms of AS.

Some examples of biologics that are used to treat AS include:

1. Tumour necrosis factor-alpha (TNF-alpha) inhibitors: These drugs, such as infliximab, adalimumab, and etanercept, work by blocking the action of TNF-alpha, which is a key molecule involved in inflammation.

2. Interleukin-17 (IL-17) inhibitors: These drugs, such as secukinumab and Ixekizumab, work by blocking the activity of IL-17,

which is another important molecule involved in inflammation.
3. Interleukin-23 (IL-23) inhibitors: These drugs, such as ustek-
   inumab, work by blocking the activity of IL-23, which is involved
   in the activation of immune cells that contribute to inflammation.

For me, this treatment was a lifesaver. It enabled me to return to a degree of normality in life. While these treatments will not stop the disease nor is a cure, the hope is that they will slow the progression. This was important for my mental stability, for some time I could escape that perpetual roundabout of AS. It is important to understand like many drugs your body could become immune to the drugs and there could, like in my case a period of regression where the drugs no longer work. Hope is not lost though, as there are many different types of biological treatments to change to. It is worthwhile mentioning if you also have any form of cancer, then the choice of treatment will be reduced as I have covered.

Biological therapies are medications that are designed to target specific components of the immune system to treat various diseases, including autoimmune disorders, cancer, and other conditions. As with any medication, biological therapies can cause side effects, which may vary depending on the individual and the specific medication being used.

Some common side effects of biological therapy may include:

1. Injection site reactions: Many biological therapies are admin-
   istered by injection, and injection site reactions, such as pain,
   swelling, and redness, are common.
2. Flu-like symptoms: Some biological therapies can cause flu-like
   symptoms, such as fever, chills, fatigue, and muscle aches.
3. Nausea and vomiting: Some individuals may experience nausea

and vomiting after receiving biological therapy.

4. Diarrhoea: Some biological therapies can cause diarrhoea or other digestive issues.
5. Skin reactions: Some biological therapies can cause skin reactions, such as rashes, itching, or dryness.
6. Increased risk of infections: Biological therapies can suppress the immune system, which can increase the risk of infections.
7. Blood pressure changes: Some biological therapies can cause changes in blood pressure, which may need to be monitored.

It's important to note that not all individuals will experience these side effects, and some may experience other side effects that are not listed here. If you are receiving biological therapy and are experiencing side effects, it's important to speak with your healthcare provider for guidance on managing symptoms and any necessary monitoring or treatment.

Who can be affected by AS

AS can affect anyone, regardless of age, gender, or ethnicity, although it tends to develop in early adulthood and is more common in men than women.

AS is a genetic condition, meaning that it can be passed down through families. However, not everyone who has the gene associated with AS will develop the condition. Only a small percentage of people with the gene will develop the disease, suggesting that other factors, such as environmental triggers, may also be involved.

AS can also be associated with other conditions, such as inflammatory bowel disease, psoriasis, and uveitis (an inflammation of the eye).

Therefore, people who have these conditions may also be at a higher risk of developing AS.

The symptoms of AS can vary widely from person to person, and it can be difficult to diagnose because it often develops gradually and progresses slowly. However, there are some common signs and symptoms that may indicate the presence of AS, including:

1. Pain and stiffness in the lower back, hips, and buttocks that is worse in the morning or after prolonged periods of sitting or standing.
2. Pain and stiffness that improves with exercise or movement.
3. Fatigue and weakness.
4. Reduced flexibility in the spine and other joints.
5. Swelling and tenderness in the affected joints.
6. Eye inflammation (uveitis) in some cases.

If you are experiencing these symptoms, it's important to see a doctor, ideally a rheumatologist, who specializes in arthritis and other musculoskeletal conditions. The doctor may perform a physical exam, take a medical history, and order diagnostic tests, such as X-rays, MRI, or blood tests, to help diagnose AS and rule out other conditions with similar symptoms. Early diagnosis and treatment are essential to prevent further damage and improve quality of life. I was asked to have a blood test to see if I was positive for AS. The blood test will show if you are positive for the HLA-B27 Gene.

<u>What is an HLA-B27 Gene</u>

HLA-B27 is a gene that provides instructions for making a protein called a human leukocyte antigen (HLA) class I molecule. HLA molecules play a critical role in the immune system by presenting foreign substances, such as viruses or bacteria, to immune cells for recognition and destruction.

HLA-B27 is a specific variant of the HLA class I molecule that is found on the surface of many types of cells in the body, including white blood cells and joint cells. HLA-B27 is associated with an increased risk of developing certain autoimmune diseases, such as ankylosing spondylitis (AS), reactive arthritis, psoriatic arthritis, and inflammatory bowel disease (IBD).

However, it's important to note that having the HLA-B27 gene does not necessarily mean that a person will develop one of these conditions, as many people with the gene do not develop any symptoms. It's believed that other factors, such as environmental triggers, may be involved in the development of these conditions in people who carry the gene.

What Triggers the HLA-B27 Gene

The exact triggers of the HLA-B27 gene are not fully understood, but it is believed that a combination of genetic and environmental factors are involved in the development of conditions associated with the gene, such as ankylosing spondylitis (AS) and reactive arthritis.

Some environmental factors that have been implicated in triggering the HLA-B27 gene and promoting the development of AS and other conditions include:

1. Infections: Certain bacterial or viral infections have been associated with the onset of reactive arthritis, which shares many

symptoms with AS.

2. Gut microbiota: There is evidence that suggests the composition of the gut microbiome may play a role in triggering autoimmune responses in people with HLA-B27.

3. Stress: Psychological stress has been linked to the development of autoimmune diseases, including AS.

4. Environmental toxins: Exposure to certain environmental toxins, such as heavy metals, may contribute to the development of AS.

It's important to note that not everyone with the HLA-B27 gene will develop AS or another associated condition, and the exact triggers may vary from person to person. Additionally, while these factors may contribute to the development of the disease, they are not the sole cause of the condition.

Links with AS and Crohn's Disease

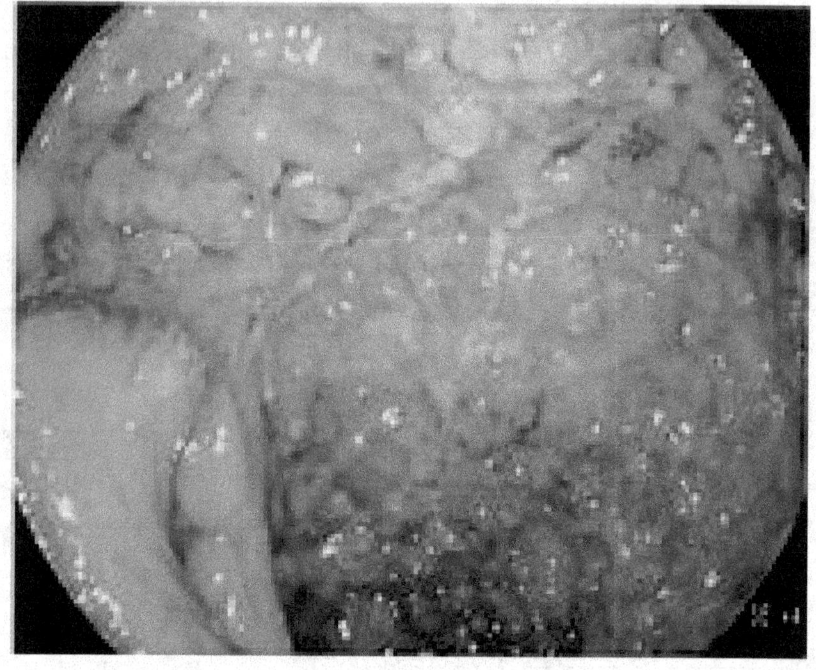

Affected Colon

There is a known association between ankylosing spondylitis (AS) and Crohn's disease, which is a type of inflammatory bowel disease (IBD). Both conditions are autoimmune diseases that involve chronic inflammation, and they share some common genetic and environmental risk factors.

Studies have shown that people with AS are more likely to develop Crohn's disease, and vice versa, compared to the general population. Up to 10% of people with AS may also have Crohn's disease and vice versa.

One possible explanation for this association is that both conditions share some common genetic factors. For example, the HLA-B27 gene, which is associated with an increased risk of developing AS, has also been linked to an increased risk of developing Crohn's disease.

Another possible explanation is that the chronic inflammation associated with these conditions may contribute to the development of the other. For example, inflammation in the gut associated with Crohn's disease may trigger inflammation in other parts of the body, including the joints and spine, leading to the development of AS.

It's important to note that while there is an association between AS and Crohn's disease, not everyone with one condition will develop the other, and the exact relationship between the two conditions is not fully understood. This was the case within my family genetics, as Crohn's was a very familiar demon within my family, where a number of my close family suffered from this debilitating disease.

<u>Links with AS and Sarcoidosis</u>

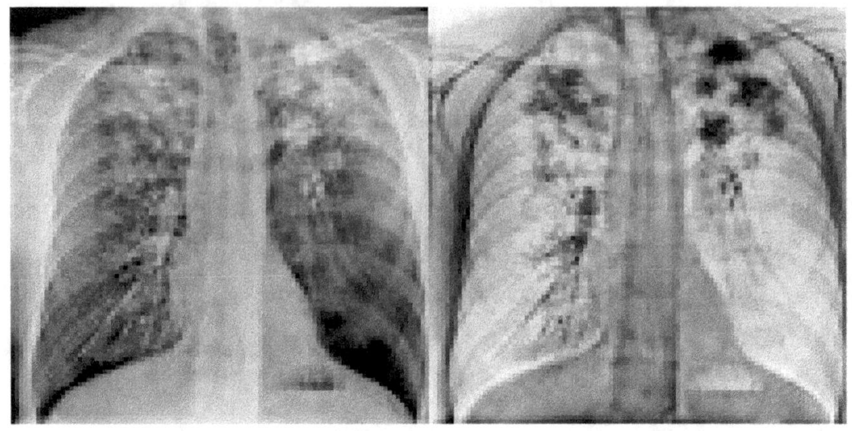

Sarcoidosis In The Lungs

Sarcoidosis is a multisystem inflammatory disease that can affect various organs in the body, including the lungs, skin, eyes, and lymph nodes. It is characterized by the formation of small clusters of inflammatory cells, called granulomas, in affected organs.

The exact cause of sarcoidosis is not fully understood, but it is believed to be an autoimmune disorder in which the immune system mistakenly attacks healthy tissue. It is also thought that environmental factors, such as exposure to certain chemicals or allergens, may play a role in triggering the disease.

Sarcoidosis can affect people of any age, gender, or ethnicity, but it is more common in adults between the ages of 20 and 40 and people of African or Scandinavian descent. The symptoms of sarcoidosis can vary widely depending on which organs are affected but may include cough, shortness of breath, chest pain, skin rashes, joint pain, and fatigue.

Sarcoidosis is typically diagnosed through a combination of medical history, physical examination, imaging tests, and laboratory tests. Treatment may involve medications to suppress the immune system and reduce inflammation, as well as supportive care to manage symptoms and improve quality of life. In many cases, sarcoidosis goes into remission on its own, but some people may experience long-term complications, such as chronic lung disease, eye damage, or neurological problems.

There is a possible association between ankylosing spondylitis (AS) and sarcoidosis, although the relationship between the two conditions is not well understood.

Sarcoidosis is a multisystem inflammatory disease that can affect various organs in the body, including the lungs, skin, and eyes. It is believed to be an autoimmune disorder, although the exact cause is unknown.

Several studies have suggested a possible link between AS and sarcoidosis. For example, one study found that people with AS were more likely to have a positive blood test for a protein called angiotensin-converting enzyme (ACE), which is often elevated in people with sarcoidosis. Other studies have found that people with AS may be more likely to develop sarcoidosis compared to the general population.

The exact relationship between the two conditions is not clear, and more research is needed to understand the underlying mechanisms. It is possible that the chronic inflammation associated with AS may contribute to the development of sarcoidosis, or that they share some common genetic or environmental risk factors. However, it's important to note that the association between AS and sarcoidosis is relatively rare, and most people with AS do not develop sarcoidosis. Ankylosing spondylitis (AS), Crohn's disease, and sarcoidosis are all autoimmune disorders that involve chronic inflammation in different parts of the body.

AS primarily affects the joints and spine, causing pain, stiffness, and limited mobility. Crohn's disease is a type of inflammatory bowel disease that affects the digestive tract, causing symptoms such as abdominal pain, diarrhoea, and weight loss. Sarcoidosis is a multisystem inflammatory disease that can affect various organs in the body, including the lungs, skin, eyes, and lymph nodes.

While the exact relationship between the three conditions is not fully understood, there is some evidence to suggest that they may share common genetic and environmental risk factors. For example, the HLA-B27 gene, which is associated with an increased risk of developing AS, has also been linked to an increased risk of developing Crohn's disease. Similarly, certain environmental factors, such as exposure to allergens or toxins, may contribute to the development of all three conditions.

It's important to note that while there may be some overlap in the underlying mechanisms of AS, Crohn's disease, and sarcoidosis, they are distinct conditions that require different treatments and management strategies. If you have been diagnosed with any of these conditions, it's essential to work closely with your healthcare provider to develop a personalized treatment plan that addresses your specific needs and symptoms.

So why have I linked these conditions together? In my research, these conditions came up time and time again, as being in the same family. While very independently different conditions, there is supporting evidence to suggest a connection with all three diseases as I have outlined.

It is also worthwhile mentioning conditions that can mimic AS or be confused with AS. As I have mentioned AS can be a very difficult disease to diagnose.

Ankylosing spondylitis (AS) can be difficult to diagnose because its symptoms may overlap with those of other conditions. Some conditions that can be mistaken for AS include:

1. Mechanical back pain: This is the most common condition that is mistaken for AS. It is caused by wear and tear on the spine due to ageing, injury, or poor posture. Unlike AS, mechanical back pain is not associated with inflammation.

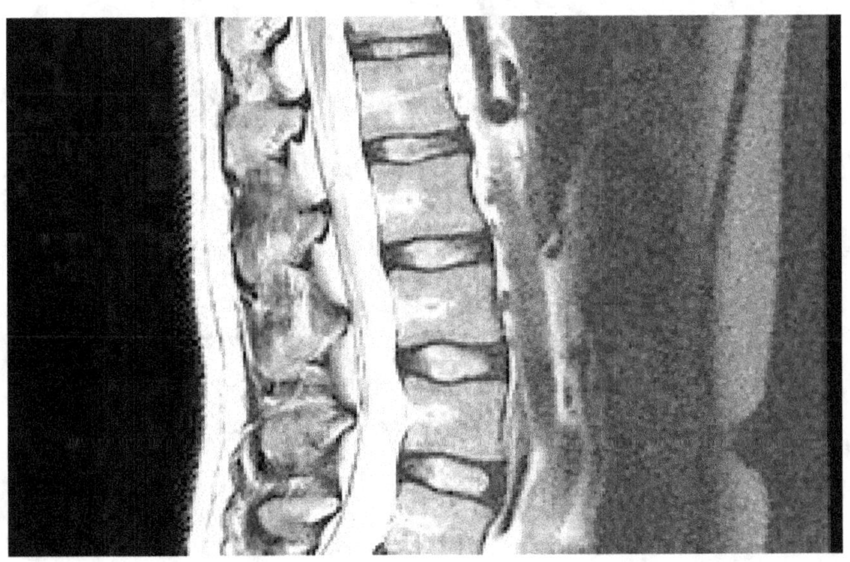

Mechanical back pain

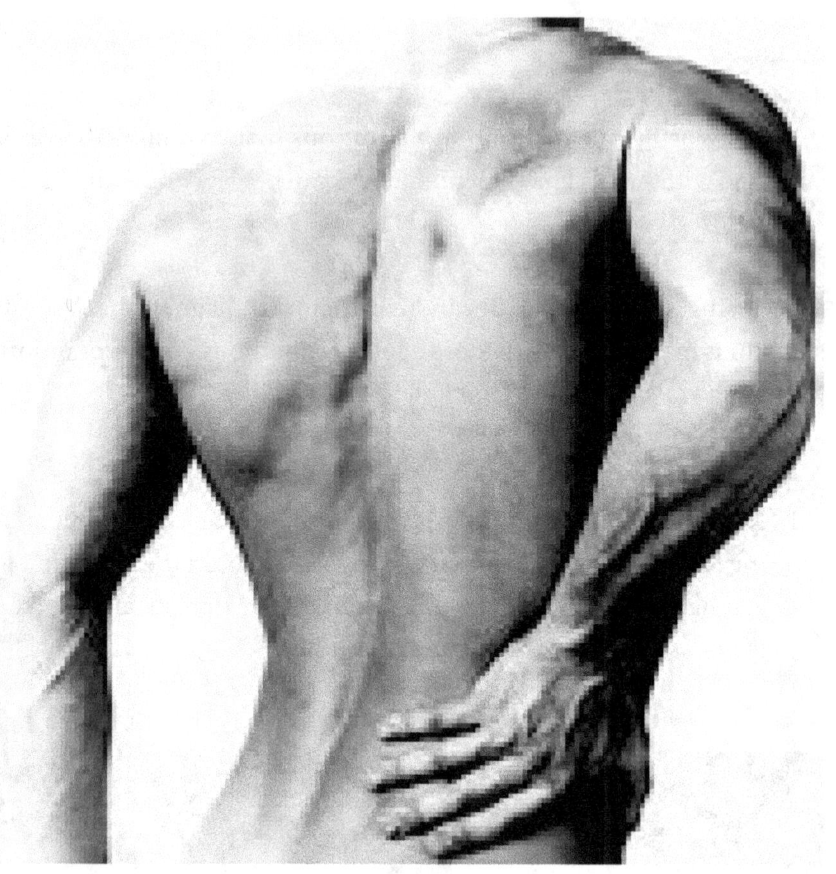

Mechanical back pain

1. Fibromyalgia: This is a condition characterized by widespread pain and tenderness in the muscles and soft tissues. Like AS, it can cause fatigue and sleep disturbances, but it does not involve joint inflammation or stiffness.

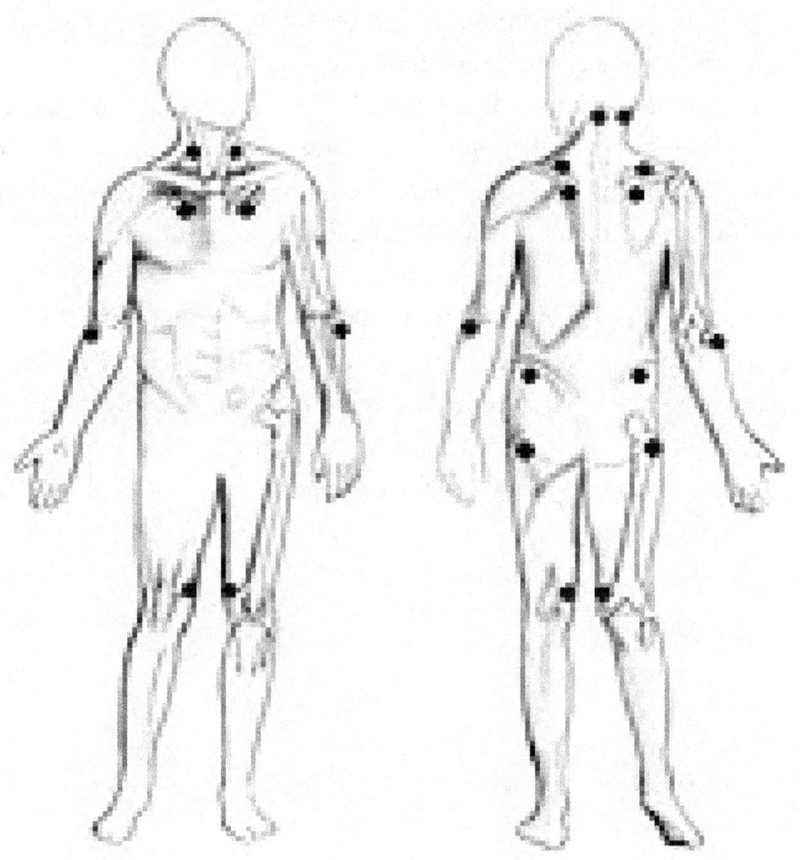

Fibromyalgia Areas

1. Psoriatic arthritis: This is a type of arthritis that can cause joint pain, stiffness, and swelling, similar to AS. It is often associated with the skin condition psoriasis, which can help distinguish it from AS.
2. Reactive arthritis: This is a type of arthritis that can develop after an infection, such as a sexually transmitted infection or a

gastrointestinal infection. It can cause joint pain and inflammation, as well as other symptoms similar to AS.

3. Inflammatory bowel disease (IBD): This includes Crohn's disease and ulcerative colitis, which are conditions that can cause inflammation in the digestive tract. They may also cause symptoms similar to AS, such as abdominal pain and diarrhoea.

If you are experiencing symptoms that may be related to AS, it's important to see a healthcare provider for an accurate diagnosis. A thorough medical history, physical examination, imaging tests, and laboratory tests can help distinguish AS from other conditions and ensure that you receive appropriate treatment.

5

What is it like living with AS?

The pain associated with ankylosing spondylitis (AS) can vary widely depending on the individual and the severity of the condition. Some common characteristics of AS pain include:

1. Low back pain: AS typically causes pain and stiffness in the lower back, which may be described as a dull ache or throbbing sensation. The pain may be worse in the morning or after periods of inactivity and may improve with exercise or movement.
2. Pain in the hips and shoulders: AS can also cause pain and stiffness in the hips and shoulders, which may make it difficult to perform everyday activities such as lifting or reaching.
3. Pain in the chest: In some cases, AS can cause pain and tightness in the chest, which may be mistaken for a heart attack.
4. Pain in the buttocks: AS can cause pain and stiffness in the buttocks, which may be more severe on one side than the other.
5. Pain in other joints: In some cases, AS can cause pain and inflammation in other joints, such as the knees, ankles, and wrists.

It's important to note that AS pain is often accompanied by stiffness, which may be worse in the morning or after periods of inactivity. The pain and stiffness may improve with exercise or movement but may worsen with rest or inactivity. If you are experiencing persistent pain or stiffness, it's important to see a healthcare provider for an accurate diagnosis and appropriate treatment.

In my experience, I have suffered from a lot of systems as I have outlined that can come and go at any time. In addition, my disease has progressed to some deformity around my upper neck with a C7 compression, restricting movement in my head movement resulting in pain when moving my head or looking over my shoulder.

I have experience exostosis in my elbow that is extremely painful with movement and lifting objects.

Exostosis is a medical term that refers to the development of new bone growth on the surface of an existing bone. This condition is also known as osteoma or bone spur. Exostosis can occur in any part of the body, but it is most common in the bones of the hands, feet, knees, and spine.

Exostosis is usually painless and does not cause any symptoms. However, if the bony growths are located near a joint or nerve, they may cause pain, swelling, and reduced range of motion. In some cases, exostosis can also cause deformities or disfigurement.

Exostosis can be caused by a variety of factors, including genetic predisposition, trauma or injury to the bone, or chronic inflammation. Treatment for exostosis depends on the severity of the condition and the location of the bony growths. In some cases, no treatment is necessary. However, if the growths are causing pain or other symptoms, they may need to be surgically removed. Physical therapy, medication, or other treatments may also be recommended to manage symptoms and improve mobility.

There is no definitive cure for exostosis, as it is a structural change in the bone. However, treatment may be recommended to manage symptoms, improve mobility, and prevent complications. Treatment options for exostosis may include:

1. Observation: If the bony growths are small and not causing any symptoms, no treatment may be necessary. The growths can be monitored over time to ensure that they are not growing or causing any complications.
2. Pain management: If the bony growths are causing pain or discomfort, over-the-counter pain medications, such as acetaminophen or nonsteroidal anti-inflammatory drugs (NSAIDs), may be recommended to manage symptoms.
3. Physical therapy: Exercises and stretches can help improve range of motion and strength, as well as relieve pain and discomfort.
4. Surgery: In some cases, surgical removal of the bony growths may be necessary if they are causing significant pain or interfering with normal movement. Surgery may also be recommended if the growths are located near a joint or nerve and are causing nerve compression or other complications.

It's important to note that treatment for exostosis depends on the location and severity of the growth, as well as the individual's symptoms and overall health. If you are experiencing pain, swelling, or other symptoms related to exostosis, it's important to see a healthcare provider for an accurate diagnosis and appropriate treatment recommendations.

6

My Cancer

As I have covered in Living with AS, in 2019 I was diagnosed with Prostrate Cancer, at fifty-five years old. I was told it was not common at my age to have prostrate cancer unless a close member of your family had been diagnosed with this type of cancer before, father or brother.

Again, like my AS diagnoses, prostate cancer is not fast-growing cancer, and if caught in time, is one of the more curable cancers. While I was diagnosed in 2019, we can turn the clock back many years in hindsight and examine the changes in my body I experienced.

Some of the details may appear personal; however, I feel it is important to cover the changes which are indicators that something may be wrong. One thing I have realised over the years is how your body speaks to you, now that might sound a bit strange to say, but there is no one knows our bodies as we do. If we cut our finger, it hurts, and it will bleed, likewise if there is a problem internally our bodies will tell us.

Overall, the body has a sophisticated system for detecting and responding to threats or abnormalities, which involves various signalling pathways and feedback mechanisms. This system helps to maintain homeostasis, or balance, in the body, and to protect against illness, injury, and disease.

It is important to state, prostate problems do not always indicate that you have cancer.

An enlarged prostate, also known as benign prostatic hyperplasia (BPH), is a common condition that affects many men as they age. The prostate gland is a small gland located beneath the bladder, and it produces fluid that helps to nourish and protect sperm.

As men age, the prostate gland can enlarge, which can cause various symptoms, such as:

1. Increased frequency of urination
2. Difficulty starting urination
3. Weak urine stream
4. Incomplete emptying of the bladder
5. Dribbling at the end of urination
6. Urinary tract infections

The exact cause of BPH is not fully understood, but it is believed to be related to changes in hormone levels as men age. Testosterone, a male hormone, is converted to dihydrotestosterone (DHT) in the prostate gland, which can contribute to the growth of prostate cells.

Treatment for an enlarged prostate may include medications, such as alpha-blockers or 5-alpha reductase inhibitors, which can help to improve urinary symptoms. In some cases, surgery may be necessary to remove or reduce the size of the prostate gland.

If you are experiencing symptoms of an enlarged prostate, it's important to speak with your doctor for an accurate diagnosis and appropriate treatment recommendations.

Perhaps if I had applied the same thinking process to my Prostate cancer as I did with my AS I may not be in the position I am in with my cancer.

The forgiveness I offer myself is, I was already dealing with a life-changing disease with AS, so less willing to admit or accept that indeed I may have another life-changing disease.

What is Prostate Cancer?

Prostate cancer is a type of cancer that occurs in the prostate, a small walnut-shaped gland in men that produces the seminal fluid that nourishes and transports sperm. Prostate cancer is one of the most common types of cancer in men, and it is estimated that 1 in 9 men will be diagnosed with prostate cancer during their lifetime. Prostate cancer usually grows slowly and initially remains confined to the prostate gland, where it may not cause serious harm. However, while some types of prostate cancer grow slowly and may need minimal or no treatment, other types are aggressive and can spread quickly.

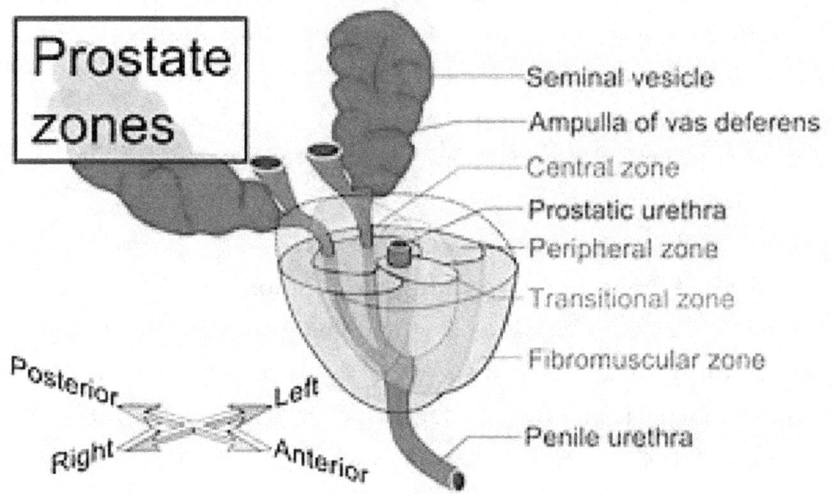

Outline Of The Prostrate

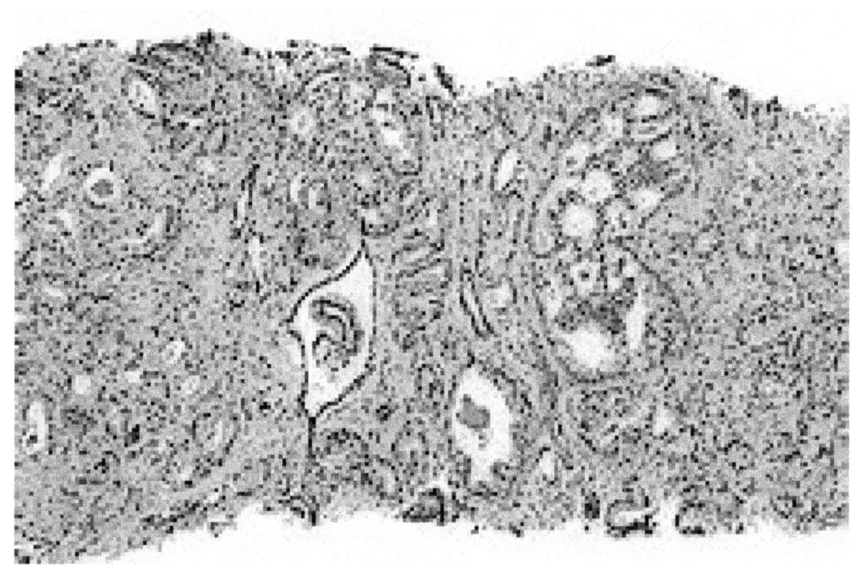

Cancer Cells Present Within The Prostrate

The exact cause of prostate cancer is unknown, but certain risk factors have been identified, including age, family history, ethnicity, and diet. Treatment options for prostate cancer include surgery, radiation therapy, hormone therapy, chemotherapy, immunotherapy, and targeted therapy.

Symptoms of Prostrate Cancer and Classification?

Prostate cancer is classified as a malignant tumour, meaning it is a cancerous growth that can spread to other parts of the body. It is typically categorized into four stages: localized (stage I and II), locally advanced (stage III), and metastatic (stage IV). The stage of prostate cancer is determined by factors such as the size of the tumour, whether it has spread to nearby lymph nodes, bones or other organs, and the Gleason score. This can cause pain, difficulty urinating, and other symptoms.

It can be seen as

Localized Prostate Cancer Localized prostate cancer is confined to the prostate gland and has not spread to other parts of the body. This type of prostate cancer can be treated with surgery, radiation therapy, or active surveillance (watchful waiting).

Advanced Prostate Cancer Advanced prostate cancer has spread beyond the prostate gland to other parts of the body. Treatment options for advanced prostate cancer include hormone therapy, chemotherapy, immunotherapy, and targeted therapy.

What is a Gleason Score

The Gleason score is a system used to grade prostate cancer. It is based on the microscopic appearance of a prostate biopsy and ranges from 2 to 10, with higher numbers indicating more aggressive cancer. The Gleason score is an important factor in determining the stage and prognosis of prostate cancer. Gleason score is only one factor to be considered when looking at the different stages of prostate cancer, and should not be focused as the primary indicator.

7

Let's Examine My Case.

our years before my diagnosis in 2019, I started to notice changes in my sexual function. Occasionally I would suffer from erectile dysfunction, but let's face it, what guy has not suffered from ED at some point in their life? Unless you are in your teens or early twenties of course.

At first, I did not think much about it, I had no reason to, I put it down to working hard, or burning the proverbial candle at both ends. As time marched on I started to notice my ED became more frequent, I might have been able to achieve an erection but had difficulty maintaining it. I had no reason to be concerned as my research always pointed to it being one of those things that can come and go especially as you get older.

That was to one day I thought I noticed blood in my urine, to be honest, I could not be sure if that was the case so I just forgot about it as most men do, burring my head in the sand so to speak. A few months passed and it happened again, but a little more pronounced, again I thought I was healthy; therefore no reason to have blood in my urine, perhaps this time it was something I ate or too many glasses of red wine. Always looking for that rational explanation as to why it was.

Some time passed again, and then the hammer blow, I had blood in my semen, which was an internal game changer for me. This did grab my attention, but why? I was healthy no reason to worry, this was what I kept telling myself. I was back to burying my head in the sand. There was no consistency to what I was experiencing, so it was one of those things, right?

Wrong, it happened again a month later; however, there was a lot more blood this time, I am sure we all have had that moment when you think ohh shit this is a problem. Not for one minute did I connect this issue could be a problem with my prostate? I knew I had to pull my head out of the sand and go to my general practitioner (GP). Like all strong or not-so-strong men, we internalise what is happing with our bodies, we convince all will be fine and it will go away on its own.

I made my appointment with my GP, just hoping she was not going to ask me to take my pants off and certainly not stick two fingers anywhere it's not meant to go, you men know what I mean lol. For those that may not know what is involved in a prostate exam.

During a prostate exam, your doctor will insert a gloved, lubricated finger into the rectum to feel the prostate gland. This allows the doctor to check for any abnormalities or signs of prostate problems, such as an enlarged prostate or lumps, this can be uncomfortable or embarrassing for some men, but it is a simple and important procedure for maintaining prostate health. Prostate cancer, for example, often has no symptoms in its early stages, so a prostate exam can help to detect it early and improve treatment outcomes. Prostate exams are typically recommended for men starting at age 50, or earlier if there is a family history of prostate problems or other risk factors.

To my joy when I explained what had been happening to my GP, there was no need to remove my pants, she said it was one of those things! It happens, it's like a nosebleed down there. A blood vessel bursts and leave the body via urine or seamen. To my delight, she said she would not subject me to the unpleasant experience of a prostrate exam.

I skipped out of her office safe in the knowledge all was and all will be just fine, just what we men want to hear. All was well in the world. Wrong!! The following afternoon I had a call from my GP stating I need to see you tomorrow. She mentioned she had been speaking with a college in the US and had been explaining my symptoms, he felt I need further investigatory follow-up to rule out anything more sinister.

So my world was back in a spin again, relief of nothing being wrong was very short-lived indeed. I had an appointment for the following day, and my worst fears were realised, I was asked to remove my pants and these fingers were indeed going to go somewhere very unpleasant. Just pull your knees up and breathe deeply she said, as my examination started, It felt like I was going to pass a brick from my rear end. I am sure the men out there that had this examination done can relate to the picture I am painting.

She explained that my prostate felt smooth, not enlarged with no lumps or bumps, it was a good sign, maybe after all it was just one of those things. She took some blood to be on the safe side to test my PSA Levels, but she was very confident 99% sure all blood tests would come back negative for cancer markers. I was not in any of the risk categories, and I had no family history of prostate cancer with my father or brothers.

The most common blood marker used to detect prostate cancer is the prostate-specific antigen (PSA) test. PSA is a protein produced by the cells of the prostate gland and can be detected in a man's blood. Elevated levels of PSA may indicate the presence of prostate cancer, although other conditions such as an enlarged prostate or prostatitis can also cause elevated PSA levels. Other blood markers that may be used to detect prostate cancer include free PSA, human kallikrein-2 (hK2), and PCA3.

Wrong again! My blood tests came back with elevated PSA levels at 3.2 indicating the possibility of prostate cancer. There was also a chance it could be prostatitis, as she previously had ruled out an enlarged prostate. The only way to be sure was to have an MRI, which had been scheduled for a couple of months out. In this situation, it is always the what-ifs and that is the hardest to deal with in my experience. I am a positive person, however; you do think about what will happen if the what-if comes out to be positive. What will happen, how bad will it be? What treatment will I need?

Four years before my diagnosis in 2019, I started to notice changes in my sexual function. Occasionally I would suffer from erectile dysfunction, but let's face it, what guy has not suffered from ED at some point in their life? Unless you are in your teens or early twenties of course.

At first, I did not think much about it, I had no reason to, I put it down to working hard, or burning the proverbial candle at both ends. As time marched on I started to notice my ED became more frequent, I might have been able to achieve an erection but had difficulty maintaining it. I had no reason to be concerned as my research always pointed to it being one of those things that can come and go especially as you get older.

That was to one day I thought I noticed blood in my urine, to be honest, I could not be sure if that was the case so I just forgot about it as most men do, burring my head in the sand so to speak. A few months passed and it happened again, but a little more pronounced, again I thought I was healthy; therefore no reason to have blood in my urine, perhaps this time it was something I ate or too many glasses of red wine. Always looking for that rational explanation as to why it was.

Some time passed again, and then the hammer blow, I had blood in my semen, which was an internal game changer for me. This did grab my attention, but why? I was healthy no reason to worry, this was what I kept telling myself. I was back to burying my head in the sand. There was no consistency to what I was experiencing, so it was one of those things, right?

Wrong, it happened again a month later; however, there was a lot more blood this time, I am sure we all have had that moment when you think ohh shit this is a problem. Not for one minute did I connect this issue could be a problem with my prostate? I knew I had to pull my head out of the sand and go to my general practitioner (GP). Like all strong or not-so-strong men, we internalise what is happing with our bodies, we convince all will be fine and it will go away on its own.

I made my appointment with my GP, just hoping she was not going to ask me to take my pants off and certainly not stick two fingers anywhere it's not meant to go, you men know what I mean lol. For those that may not know what is involved in a prostate exam.

During a prostate exam, your doctor will insert a gloved, lubricated finger into the rectum to feel the prostate gland. This allows the doctor to check for any abnormalities or signs of prostate problems, such as an enlarged prostate or lumps, this can be uncomfortable or embarrassing for some men, but it is a simple and important procedure for maintaining prostate health. Prostate cancer, for example, often has no symptoms in its early stages, so a prostate exam can help to detect it early and improve treatment outcomes. Prostate exams are typically recommended for men starting at age 50, or earlier if there is a family history of prostate problems or other risk factors.

To my joy when I explained what had been happening to my GP, there was no need to remove my pants, she said it was one of those things! It happens, it's like a nosebleed down there. A blood vessel bursts and leave the body via urine or seamen. To my delight, she said she would not subject me to the unpleasant experience of a prostrate exam.

I skipped out of her office safe in the knowledge all was and all will be just fine, just what we men want to hear. All was well in the world. Wrong!! The following afternoon I had a call from my GP stating I need to see you tomorrow. She mentioned she had been speaking with a college in the US and had been explaining my symptoms, he felt I need further investigatory follow-up to rule out anything more sinister.

So my world was back in a spin again, relief of nothing being wrong was very short-lived indeed. I had an appointment for the following day, and my worst fears were realised, I was asked to remove my pants and these fingers were indeed going to go somewhere very unpleasant. Just pull your knees up and breathe deeply she said, as my examination started, It felt like I was going to pass a brick from my rear end. I am sure the men out there that had this examination done can relate to the picture I am painting.

She explained that my prostate felt smooth, not enlarged with no lumps or bumps, it was a good sign, maybe after all it was just one of those things. She took some blood to be on the safe side to test my PSA Levels, but she was very confident 99% sure all blood tests would come back negative for cancer markers. I was not in any of the risk categories, and I had no family history of prostate cancer with my father or brothers.

The most common blood marker used to detect prostate cancer is the prostate-specific antigen (PSA) test. PSA is a protein produced by the cells of the prostate gland and can be detected in a man's blood. Elevated levels of PSA may indicate the presence of prostate cancer, although other conditions such as an enlarged prostate or prostatitis can also cause elevated PSA levels. Other blood markers that may be used to detect prostate cancer include free PSA, human kallikrein-2 (hK2), and PCA3.

Wrong again! My blood tests came back with elevated PSA levels at 3.2 indicating the possibility of prostate cancer. There was also a chance it could be prostatitis, as she previously had ruled out an enlarged prostate. The only way to be sure was to have an MRI, which had been scheduled for a couple of months out. In this situation, it is always the what-ifs and that is the hardest to deal with in my experience. I am a positive person, however; you do think about what will happen if the what-if comes out to be positive. What will happen, how bad will it be? What treatment will I need?

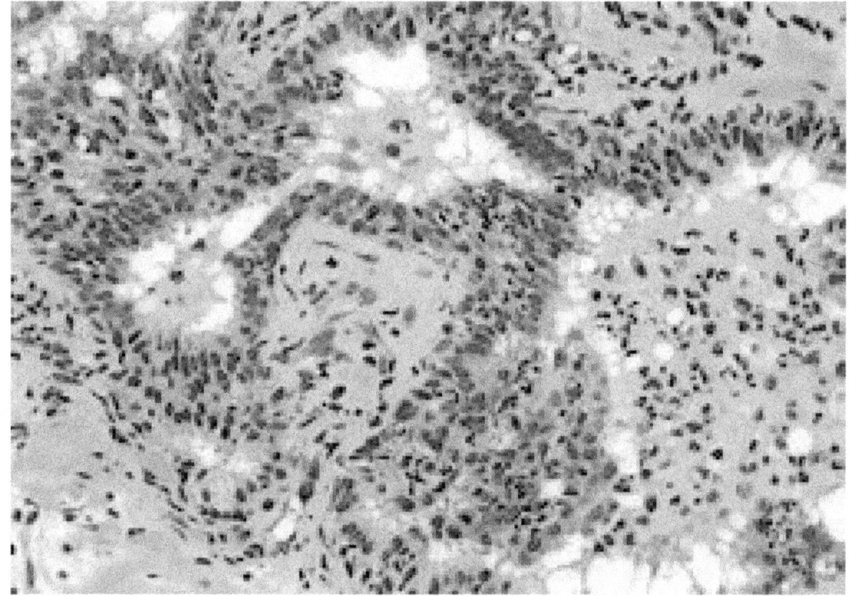

Prostatitis

Prostatitis is an inflammation of the prostate gland, It can be caused by bacterial infection, physical injury, or stress. Symptoms of prostatitis include pain in the lower abdomen or pelvic area, difficulty urinating, and frequent urination. Treatment for prostatitis may include antibiotics, anti-inflammatory medications, lifestyle changes, and other therapies.

My time comes around for my MRI, still, all the what-if swimming around in my head, after you are back into the waiting game for the results of the MRI which can take up to six weeks for reporting.

My concerns were confirmed, indeed I had a prostate cancer lesion on the right lobe, to grade cancer will require biopsies to be taken, not the waiting intensives as now I know but don't know the grade and size. Stress levels 100%.

Biopsies were taken, and I would like to say, not downgrading the pain of childbirth at all, under local pain relief it was right up there lol. Results are in presenting PSA 4.8 so have gone up, and my Gleason score of 6. Pretty conclusive that I have prostate cancer.

What Does a Gleason Score Mean?

Gleason score 6 is a prostate cancer grading system used to determine the aggressiveness of a tumour. It is based on the pattern of cells seen under a microscope and ranges from 2-10, with higher numbers indicating more aggressive tumours. A Gleason score of 6 indicates that the tumour is moderately differentiated and has an intermediate risk of progression.

Treatment Discussion and Careplan.

In my opinion, this is where my treatment plan starts to unravel, and perhaps not given the importance it required for intermediate risk of progression.

Intermediate-risk prostate cancer is a form of the disease that is more advanced than low-risk prostate cancer but not as severe as high-risk prostate cancer. Intermediate-risk prostate cancer typically has a Gleason score of 7 or higher, meaning that the cancer cells are more aggressive and likely to spread beyond the prostate gland.

Treatment for intermediate-risk prostate cancer typically involves some combination of surgery, radiation therapy, hormone therapy, chemotherapy, or active surveillance. The exact treatment plan will depend on factors such as age, overall health, and personal preferences.

My care plan did not offer any further treatment, at the time of the results obtained. The new way of thinking was active surveillance, this was a watch-and-see process with a regular blood test to monitor your PSA for changes.

I have to be honest, this did not sit well with me, I was concerned as to the possibility of continued growth and it is missed. As it turned out my concerns were not misplaced. I did ask to see the consultant to discuss the post diagnoses care plan. I was made to feel I was questing their expert knowledge and after all, who was I?

I was told at that time, "My cancer was so small it was a push to even call it cancer, and that my AS would give me much more bother and would be more troublesome than my Prostate cancer ever would. He went on to say at my age I would die with prostate cancer and not of prostate cancer" I struggle to conceptualise how he could structure and make his determined hypothesis, as there was no medical evidence to support his statement. I would argue in this contact there was more opinion on his part than medical evidence to support his statement. In my view cancer is cancer.

Nevertheless, I was told I would not be receiving any form of treatment as of that time and will remain on active surveillance for the foreseeable future. I was to have my three monthly blood tests that will map any progression of my disease. My PSA blood tests were mapping around 4.8 to 4.9 on the face of it relatively stable, well that's what was supposed to happen.

We all know in early 2020 Covid-19 hit the world and we all went into lockdown. Many medical services were closed down, rightly to support the much-needed care for those that were sadly contracting Covid-19.

While most services were suspended, it was always possible to speak with my medical team if I felt things had changed.

I will take you back to the statements I made about knowing your own body and the inner voice we need to listen to. Over the period between 2020 and 2022, I felt that my cancer position was changing. I had an inner sense my body was telling me things are not right, I needed help. My symptoms were increasing, I was in a lot of discomfort with pain in my pubic area and rectum. I was finding it difficult to pass urine, I continually need to pass water, but never felt I was emptying my bladder. I just generally felt very unwell.

I made contact with the urology department, outlining the changes I felt had taken place. As part of the active surveillance, I was to have an MRI every eighteen months on top of the blood tests, I was overdue this by six months. After a lengthy telephone conversation. Urology Department agreed to send me for a follow-up MRI. To determine if indeed there are any further changes within my prostate and cancer site.Having waited some eight weeks for the results of the MRI. It was determined that. Indeed, there were as mild changes to my cancer, mild being to both lobes of the prostate left lobe having cancer on the apex.

If prostate cancer is located on the apex of the prostate, it may affect the function of the urethra and the ability to urinate. Depending on the size and extent of the cancerous growth, treatment options may include surgery, radiation therapy, or other therapies aimed at destroying or removing the cancerous cells. In my case, despite having mild changes as was documented it was also reported the MRI study was limited due to poor diffusion imaging, red flag to me! but it appeared not to my medical team.

Despite the poor diffusion imaging, I was informed by my consultant was more than happy to have me remain on active surveillance (wait and see) second red flag to me. Again I will underline the need to listen to our bodies and mine was telling me what I was being told did not fit with what I was being told. My PSA markers had jumped from 4.8 to 9.7 within six months again reinforcing that something was not right. Never be afraid to question your medical team, if you do not agree with what you are being told.

My medical team were very reluctant to progress with further tests following my MRI results, my concern was that things were much more progressed than I was being told. In my experience, doctors can make mistakes also and I did not want to be another static.

I pushed hard for further biopsies to determine how much my disease had progressed and I knew I would get that from understanding if my Gleason score had changed from previous biopsies. I was right to push for the right answers as my Gleason score had gone from 3+3=6 to bilateral anterior 3+4=7, I had crossed the threshold of now needing treatment. If I had listened to my medical team and remained on surveillance for a further twelve months as was suggested, I firmly believe I would have fallen into the terminal category, and that is scary.

8

Radical Robotic Prostatectomy

Given the progression of my cancer, I was limited in my options, at age 55 there was a likelihood that if my treatment was unsuccessful and could not fully be removed or returned, I need to have a plan B for the future. That being said I was only really left with one option, a radical robotic prostatectomy.

A radical robotic prostatectomy is a surgical procedure that is used to remove the entire prostate gland in men who have been diagnosed with prostate cancer. The procedure is performed using a robotic system that allows for greater precision and control during the surgery.

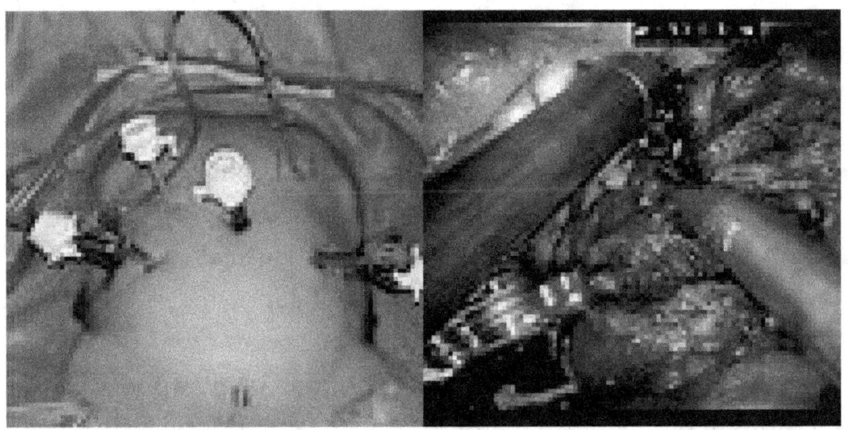

Robotic Prostatectomy

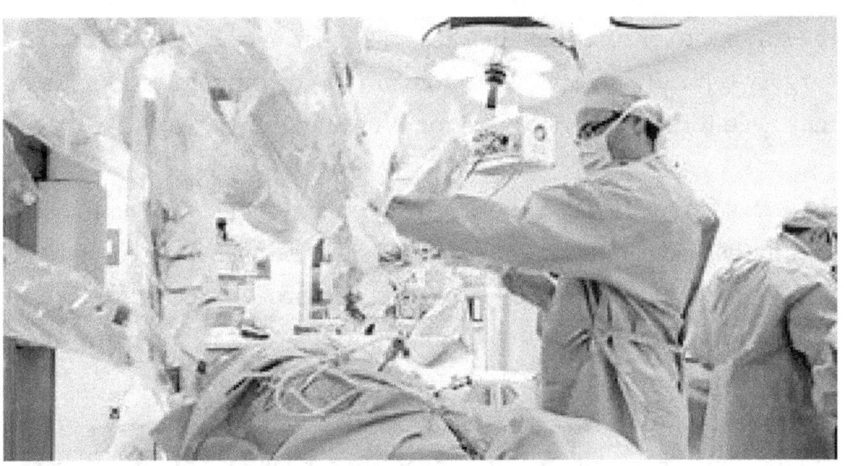

Medical Team Setting Up Robot

Given the progression of my cancer, I was limited in my options, at age 55 there was a likelihood that if my treatment was unsuccessful and could not fully be removed or returned, I need to have a plan B for the future. That being said I was only really left with one option, a radical robotic prostatectomy.

A radical robotic prostatectomy is a surgical procedure that is used to remove the entire prostate gland in men who have been diagnosed with prostate cancer. The procedure is performed using a robotic system that allows for greater precision and control during the surgery.

During a radical robotic prostatectomy, the surgeon makes small incisions in the abdomen to insert a camera and surgical instruments. The surgeon then uses a console to control the robotic arms and perform the surgery while viewing a 3D image of the surgical area.

The prostate gland and surrounding tissue are carefully removed during the surgery to ensure that all cancerous cells have been removed. The surgery typically takes three to four hours to complete, and patients may need to stay in the hospital for a few days to recover.

Recovery from a radical robotic prostatectomy can take several weeks or months, and patients may experience side effects such as pain, fatigue, and urinary incontinence. However, the procedure is effective in removing prostate cancer and improving survival rates in many men.

It's important to note that a radical robotic prostatectomy may not be the best option for all men with prostate cancer, and other treatment options may be considered depending on the stage and severity of cancer. It is important to speak with your healthcare provider for guidance on appropriate testing and treatment options for you. Always do your research before meeting your medical team and deciding on your treatment path. Ask as many questions as you need to help make the correct treatment decisions for your condition.

The day came for my surgery, 05 October 2023, I would be lying if I did not say I was apprehensive of the operation and the side effects I was going to experience in the future. The operation did not run smoothly as I would have liked, I discovered I had an intolerance to opiate, which just meant I had to stay longer in ICU, but really no big deal. I was just glad to have the operation over. It was important for my mental well-being to get through as upbeat as I could. To achieve this, I had set small milestones for after the operation. I wanted to be up and moving as soon as I could after the operation, to be able to shower myself and be self-motivating, this was how I had prepared myself to overcome the obstacles I would face.

I was discharged four days post-operation with a catheter to remain for seven days. Like all invasive operations, there were small medical issues to overcome. I developed a balder infection and a collection of blood in my pelvis (haematoma) all easily corrected with high doses of antibiotics.

Pathology and Histology Report

1. Biopsy: The urologist will collect a small tissue sample from the prostate gland using a needle biopsy. This is typically done using ultrasound guidance.
2. Tissue Preparation: The tissue sample is then sent to a pathology laboratory, where it is processed and prepared for examination under a microscope.
3. Staining: The tissue is usually stained with special dyes that highlight different structures in the tissue, making it easier for the pathologist to identify any abnormalities.
4. Microscopic Examination: The pathologist will examine the tissue sample under a microscope, looking for any signs of cancerous or

abnormal cells. They will look at the size, shape, and appearance of the cells to determine if they are normal or abnormal.

5. Grading: If cancer is present, the pathologist will also assign a grade to the cancerous cells based on how abnormal they appear. This is called the Gleason score, which ranges from 2 to 10 and helps determine the aggressiveness of cancer.

6. Reporting: The pathologist will then write a report summarizing their findings and send it back to the urologist, who will share the results with the patient.

It's important to note that a prostate biopsy is not 100% accurate, and there is always a chance that cancer may be missed. If a patient has symptoms or risk factors for prostate cancer, their doctor may recommend additional testing or monitoring even if the biopsy results are negative.

While waiting for that Histology report from your doctor, we are always hoping for a positive outcome, so we can move on with our lives. In my case, it was less clear-cut. The pathologist took six parallel slices from the apex to the base of my prostrate, the macroscopic features were prescient with two calcified lesions on the left side and 1 on the right of the prostate 2 to 3mm in dimensions. It was uncertain from the pathology if my cancer had been confined only to my prostrate. They defined my type of cancer as Adenocarcinoma.

What is Adenocarcinoma cancer?

Adenocarcinoma is a type of cancer that arises from glandular cells, which produce and secrete fluids such as mucus, hormones, or digestive enzymes. This type of cancer can occur in various organs of the body, including the lung, breasts, colon, pancreas, prostate, and others.

Adenocarcinomas are typically classified based on their location and the appearance of the cancerous cells under a microscope. For example, lung adenocarcinomas are often classified based on the pattern of growth, such as lepidic, acinar, papillary, or solid. Prostate adenocarcinomas are often classified based on their Gleason score, which reflects the degree of abnormality and aggressiveness of the cancer cells.

Adenocarcinomas can have different signs and symptoms depending on the affected organ. Some common symptoms may include unexplained weight loss, fatigue, pain or discomfort in the affected area, changes in bowel or bladder habits, or abnormal bleeding or discharge. Treatment options for adenocarcinomas depend on various factors, such as the stage and location of the cancer, the patient's overall health, and their preferences. Treatment may include surgery, radiation therapy, chemotherapy, hormone therapy, or targeted therapy.

The curability of adenocarcinoma cancer depends on various factors, such as the stage and location of cancer, the patient's overall health, and the effectiveness of the treatment. Early-stage adenocarcinomas that are confined to the primary organ and have not spread to other parts of the body may have a higher chance of cure than advanced-stage cancers that have metastasized to other organs.

For example, localized prostate adenocarcinoma, which is confined to the prostate gland, has a 5-year survival rate of nearly 100% for most men. However, metastatic prostate adenocarcinoma, which has spread to other organs such as bones, has a much lower 5-year survival rate of around 30%. Similarly, early-stage lung adenocarcinomas have a higher chance of curing than advanced-stage cancers.

Treatment options for adenocarcinoma cancer typically include surgery, radiation therapy, chemotherapy, hormone therapy, or targeted therapy. The choice of treatment depends on various factors, such as the stage and location of the cancer, the patient's overall health, and their preferences. In general, a multidisciplinary team of doctors and specialists will work together to develop an individualized treatment plan for each patient.

It's important to note that even if adenocarcinoma cancer is not curable, treatments can often help control the cancer, relieve symptoms, and improve quality of life. In some cases, cancer can be managed as a chronic disease, allowing patients to live for many years with the condition. Regular check-ups and follow-up care are important for monitoring the cancer and detecting any changes or recurrence. In my case, I was left with positive margins (cancer remaining) post-surgery, this will necessitate three monthly PSA blood testing for the remainder of my life to ensure if or when it returns we catch it early, so I have the opportunity to have further treatment.

9

So what have we understood about living with AS and Prostate Cancer?

Ankylosing spondylitis (AS) and prostate cancer are two separate health conditions that can cause significant physical and emotional challenges for those affected. While it may be difficult to see the positives in these diagnoses, there are many reasons for optimism and hope when it comes to managing these conditions.

While we know prostate cancer is two distinct medical conditions that affect different parts of the body. AS affects the spine and joints, and prostate cancer affects the prostate gland in men. Although they may seem unrelated, a positive summary can be made about how these conditions have been managed and treated in recent years.

AS is a chronic inflammatory disease that primarily affects the spine, causing pain, stiffness, and limited mobility. As we have outlined there is no cure for AS, however; there are a variety of treatment options available that can help manage symptoms and improve quality of life. These may include medications to reduce inflammation and pain, physical therapy to improve flexibility and strength, and lifestyle changes such as exercise, stress management, and a healthy diet.

One of the positive aspects of AS is that it is a well-researched and well-understood condition, with many effective treatment options available. In recent years, there have been significant advances in our understanding of the genetic and environmental factors that contribute to AS, and new treatments are continually being developed and tested. With the right combination of medical care and lifestyle changes, many people with AS can live full and active lives.

Prostate cancer is a type of cancer that develops in the prostate gland, which is located near the bladder and is responsible for producing semen. While prostate cancer is a serious diagnosis, the good news is that it is often slow-growing and can be successfully treated if caught early. Treatment options for prostate cancer may include surgery, radiation therapy, chemotherapy, hormone therapy, or a combination of these therapies.

One of the most positive aspects of prostate cancer is the availability of effective screening tests, such as the prostate-specific antigen (PSA) test and the digital rectal exam (DRE). These tests can help detect prostate cancer in its early stages when it is most treatable. Additionally, advances in medical technology have made prostate cancer surgery safer and more effective than ever before, with robotic surgery and other minimally invasive techniques reducing the risk of complications and improving outcomes.

It is important to note that having AS does not increase a person's risk of developing prostate cancer, and having prostate cancer does not increase a person's risk of developing AS. However, people with AS who are diagnosed with prostate cancer may face unique challenges in managing both conditions simultaneously. For example, some AS medications may increase the risk of prostate cancer, while others may interfere with prostate cancer treatment. People with both conditions need to work closely with their healthcare providers to develop a treatment plan that takes both conditions into account.

Despite the challenges that AS and prostate cancer can present, there are many reasons to remain positive and hopeful. With the right care and support, it is possible to manage these conditions while living a fulfilling life. Some people with AS find that the diagnosis gives them a new sense of purpose and motivation, inspiring them to take charge of their health and pursue their passions. Similarly, many people with prostate cancer find that the diagnosis helps them prioritise their health and relationships, leading to a greater appreciation for life's joys.

One of the most important factors in managing AS and prostate cancer is social support. Joining a support group or connecting with others who have experienced similar challenges can provide a sense of community and help people feel less isolated. Additionally, family and friends can play a critical role in providing emotional support and practical assistance when needed.

Ankylosing spondylitis (AS) and prostate cancer can both have a significant impact on physical functioning, but staying active is crucial for maintaining physical and mental health. Here are some tips for staying active with AS and prostate cancer:

Listen to your body: Pay attention to how your body is feeling and adjust your activity level accordingly. If you are experiencing pain or fatigue, take a break or reduce the intensity of your activity.

Find low-impact exercises: Low-impact exercises are less stressful on the joints and can help improve flexibility, strength, and endurance. Swimming, yoga, and walking are great options.

Work with a physical therapist: A physical therapist can design an exercise program tailored to your specific needs and abilities, as well as teach you proper form and technique.

Incorporate stretching into your routine: Stretching can help improve flexibility, reduce stiffness, and prevent injury. Incorporate stretching exercises into your daily routine or as part of your warm-up and cool-down before and after exercise.

Stay hydrated: Drinking plenty of water is important for maintaining joint health and reducing inflammation. Make sure to stay hydrated before, during, and after exercise.

Use assistive devices: Assistive devices, such as canes or braces, can help reduce stress on the joints and improve balance and stability.

Take breaks: It's important to take breaks throughout the day to avoid overexertion and reduce fatigue. Set a timer or use an app to remind yourself to take breaks and stretch or move around.

Focus on overall wellness: In addition to exercise, focus on overall wellness by eating a healthy diet, getting enough sleep, and managing stress. These factors can all impact physical and mental health.

Be patient and persistent: Staying active with AS and prostate cancer can be challenging, but it's important to be patient and persistent. Set achievable goals and celebrate small victories along the way. Remember that any level of activity is better than none.

10

Conclusion

While AS and prostate cancer can be challenging diagnoses, there are many reasons for optimism and hope. Advances in medical research and technology are continually improving our ability to manage these conditions, and with the right care and support, it is possible to live a healthy and fulfilling life. The key is to stay positive, stay informed, and stay connected to the people and activities that bring joy and meaning to your life.

I hope this book has gone some way to helping those that may need that knowledge and understanding of many people in the world with the same diseases as ourselves

No matter what your medical provider's opinions may be, and let us face it, that is all it is, their medical opinion. Always follow your gut feeling!! remember it is your body, listen to what it is telling you. If what your body is experiencing, conflicts with medical opinion, then become well-informed about your condition, do your research, and understand the different contributory factors or variables that may be involved with your condition, can it be linked to another issue or disease? How will this affect me in the long term?

Above all, always remember you can ask for a second opinion if you are in doubt or unhappy with what you have been told.

Leaving A Review

If you have found this book to be informative and it has helped you through a very difficult period in your life, I would really appreciate it if you would leave a review on Amazon.

11

Resources

httpsttps://www.healthline.com/health/ankylosing-spondylitis/resources-for-support

Cherney, K. (2019, February 8). *9 Resources for Ankylosing Spondylitis Support*. Healthline. https://www.healthline.com/health/ankylosing-spondylitis/resources-for-support

https://ard.bmj.com/content/61/suppl_3/iii24

Van Der Heijde, D., Braun, J., McGonagle, D., & Siegel, J. (2002). Treatment trials in ankylosing spondylitis: current and future considerations. *Annals of the Rheumatic Diseases, 61*(Supplement 3), 24iii–32. https://doi.org/10.1136/ard.61.suppl_3.iii24

https://clinicaltrials.gov/ct2/show/NCT04947579

A Study of CC-99677 in Participants With Active Ankylosing Spondylitis - Full Text View - ClinicalTrials.gov. (n.d.). https://clinicaltrials.gov/ct2/show/NCT04947579

https://nass.co.uk/

National Axial Spondyloarthritis Society, including Ankylosing Spondylitis. (2023, April 23). National Axial Spondyloarthritis Society. https://-nass.co.uk/

https://spondylitis.org/

Spondylitis Association of America. (2023, April 3). *Spondylitis Association of America | Serving the Spondyloarthritis Community.* Spondylitis Association of America - Ankylosing Spondylitis. https://spondylitis.org/Copy to clipboard

https://my.clevelandclinic.org/health/diagnostics/22087-gleason-score

Gleason Score for Prostate Cancer Staging: Grades and Treatment Options. (n.d.). Cleveland Clinic. https://my.clevelandclinic.org/health/diagnostics/22087-gleason-score